Stretching for Life

Four minute stretching routines

For health
For flexibility
For injury prevention

Benjamin Griffes, M.A., D.C.

First Edition

First Printing: March, 2002
Second Printing: December, 2002

ProStar **Publications,** Inc.

3 Church Circle, Suite 109
Annapolis, MD 21401
Phone: (800) 481-6277 • Fax: (800) 487-6277
www.prostarpublications.com
orders@prostarpublications.com

stretching4life@aol.com

www.stretching4life.com

ACKNOWLEDGEMENTS

This book evolved out of the need for me to find better ways to serve my patients. For the past ten years I have been stressing the importance of stretching as a way of preventing injuries, keeping muscles and joints flexible and relaxed, and helping my patients hold their chiropractic adjustments. For the past three years, I have been leading a stretching class every Monday night. It is to those dedicated folks who have consistently showed up, and are living testament that stretching helps keep you young, that I dedicate this book: ***Art Adams, Helen Baker, Amaris Bryer, Phil Bryer, Walter Hesse, Lura Hungerford, Maria Schneider, Don Whittemore and Linda Whittemore.***

In addition, I received valuable assistance from a number of people along the way in producing this book. This was in the areas of publishing, printing, computer programming, photography, modeling, website design, editing and inspiration. Much thanks and gratitude go to: Tracy Glynn, Ed Rigsbee, Dale Jacobs, Serene Skuro, Bill Jackson, Kathy Jackson, Luis Ujueta, John Donaldson, Sharon Butler, Art Adams, Jonathan Wilson, Del Barrett, Tim Eichenberg, the book ***The Self Publishing Manual*** by Dan Poynter, and finally, ***God Almighty***, who has blessed me in so many ways.

Lastly, I would like to thank my family for their patience and assistance as I went through this whole learning process of creating, making mistakes, revising, and the long hours of sitting, typing and editing. Take comfort, Carrie, Daniel, Robin and Dustin, I plan on writing more books.

Ben Griffes

TABLE OF CONTENTS

Introduction 5

How to use this book 6

Structure determines function 8

Muscle location chart 9

Neck stretches 10

Shoulder stretches 13

Arm and wrist stretches 17

Back stretches 20

Hips/pelvis 27

Leg and foot stretches 29

4 - Minute Stretching Routines 34

Wake-up stretches 35

Back stretches #1 36

Back stretches #2 37

Back stretches #3 38

Neck & Face 39

Office #1 40

Office #2 41

Traveling (sitting) 42

Traveling (standing) 43

Warm-up (lower body #1) 44

Warm-up (lower body #2) 45

Warm-up (upper body) 46

Appendix 47

Index 55

INTRODUCTION

When we move, muscles shorten or flex while the opposite muscles lengthen or extend. This is a normal, physiological function of movement. When the flexor contracts, the extensor relaxes, and vice versa. To illustrate this, place your hand on the top of a desk and push down. Now feel the muscles with your other hand and notice that the muscle in the back of your arm is tight (contracted.) while the muscle in the front is relaxed. If you put your hand underneath the desk and push up, you will find the opposite to be true.

When you create any restriction in the muscles and fascia (connective tissue), due to trauma, adaptive shortening, or chronic, postural overload, you will affect the functioning of the muscles and joints involved in that particular movement pattern. Certainly, nutritional deficiency and genetic inheritances may affect your flexibility, but the main contributing factor that affects the loss of flexibility appears to be *mechanical interference*.

Mechanical interference can manifest itself as a result of a temporary trauma, such as strain/sprains to your ankle, knee or back. This will create compensations elsewhere in the body that can create imbalanced posture, stiff joints and achy muscles. Only when you are able to release the restriction from the original trauma will you be able to regain your normal physiological functioning.

Stretching daily helps to overcome the tightness and restrictions you create during the day. It is not a magical solution that will work independently of the other elements of good health, like adequate sleep, proper nutrition, exercise, and proper posture. Stretching alone will not keep you pain-free and relaxed if you neglect the other areas of your life.

Have fun with these stretches. The routines are all under four minutes long and options are given for easier or harder stretching, depending upon your needs. ***Please remember, this book is just one source of information on this subject.***

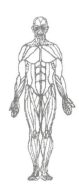

HOW TO USE THIS BOOK

This book is designed for those busy people who don't have time to stretch, for those who have difficulty stretching, and for those who don't know how to stretch. For everyone else, this book can serve as a guide for easy-to-follow stretching routines in four minutes or less.

The first half of this book shows different stretches for each area of your body (shoulders, back, etc.) which will accomplish the same stretch, but take into account any physical limitations that you might have. The second half of this book shows the stretches in four minute routines which you can use in a variety of situations.

It is always best to be warmed up prior to stretching, but some people like to use these stretches as part of their daily warm up routine. Mostly, these stretches can be done anytime during the day or evening, and certainly after you have been awake and moving for 15 to 20 minutes in the morning. You also may notice that it is easier for you to stretch after a hot shower or bath and after physical exercise.

Breathing while stretching is important because 1) you need to, and 2) it helps you to relax into the stretch. This is particularly important with very tight and stiff muscles. You will find it is easier to exhale as you increase the stretch, then inhale and hold the stretch.

Listen to your body. Stiff joints and achy muscles are telling you that you need to *move*, that you've been sitting or standing in one place for too long. Consider stretching as playtime for your muscles; something to be enjoyed, not viewed as a chore or an inconvenient necessity. Consistent stretching will assist you in feeling and looking younger. Create a lifelong habit of daily stretching. This will help you reduce the achiness and stiffness that is caused by the stress and strain common in today's society.

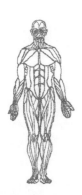

STRETCHING FOR LIFE 7

HOW TO USE THIS BOOK

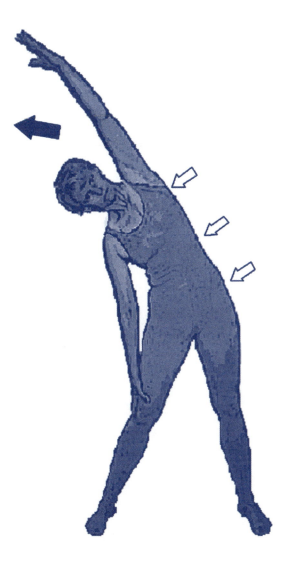

Each stretch will have a drawing and a description, telling you how to do the stretch, how long to hold it, and where you should feel the stretch. The black arrows ➡ tell you which way to move, the white arrows ⇨ tell you where you should feel the stretch.

The muscle man is shown in every section, highlighting those muscles involved in the stretches.

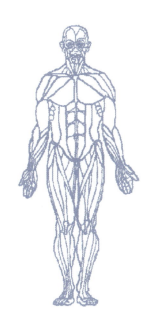

Throughout the book, italicized print will explain how or why muscles get tight, what patterns can cause you trouble, and what you can do about it.

There is often a dull, pulling feeling while stretching. If you feel a sharp pain, stop immediately, and check to see if you are doing the stretch correctly. Do it again slowly, and if the pain continues, stop, and try another stretch. If the pain continues, consult a healthcare professional.

STRUCTURE DETERMINES FUNCTION

FASCIA

Fascia is sheaths of connective tissue which are either loosely or tightly woven fibers that help muscles withstand stress and strain. Some fascia wraps around the bundles of muscle fibers while other layers of fascia wrap the whole muscle and groups of muscles. There is a fluid between the muscle and fascia which allows the freedom of movement you experience when moving. The fascia also helps hold the nerves, arteries and veins in place as they pass to and through the muscle groups.

TENDONS

The primary function of tendons is to connect muscles to bones. Tendons are made up of heavy fibers of connective tissue which can sustain forces up to 18,000 pounds per inch. Should there be excessive force, a tear will usually occur where the muscle attaches to the tendon or where the tendon attaches to the bone. Tendonitis is when the tendon becomes inflamed from trauma or dysfunction and is continually aggravated from lack of rest and rehabilitation.

LIGAMENTS

The main function of a ligament is to connect bone to bone. It is made up of thick fibers, irregular in nature, that serve to stabilize a joint. The ligaments will be located along those portions of a joint that need greater stability and limitation of movement. A sprain would be an injury to the ligaments and surrounding tissues of a joint which have been stretched or partially torn. This happens when there is excessive stress that forces a ligament beyond its maximum range of motion.

MUSCLES

Muscle fibers have the ability to contract, extend, and relax. These properties allow you to produce tension in the form of a pull or push, to lengthen and stretch, and still be able to relax and return to their original length. A muscle, along with its tendon, can be strained due to over-use, direct trauma or excessive contraction against resistance (lifting something too heavy).

NERVES

Your nervous system controls and regulates all other systems in the body. In relationship to the muscles, your movement is dependent upon muscular action, and muscular action is dependent on the nervous system. Innervation of the musculoskeletal system by the nerves provides for growth, repair, postural balance, muscle tone and joint movement. When there is nerve pressure or damage, the function of the nerve is compromised and reduced, thus affecting the growth, repair and normal function of the tissues and fibers it was meant to control.

STRETCHING FOR LIFE 9

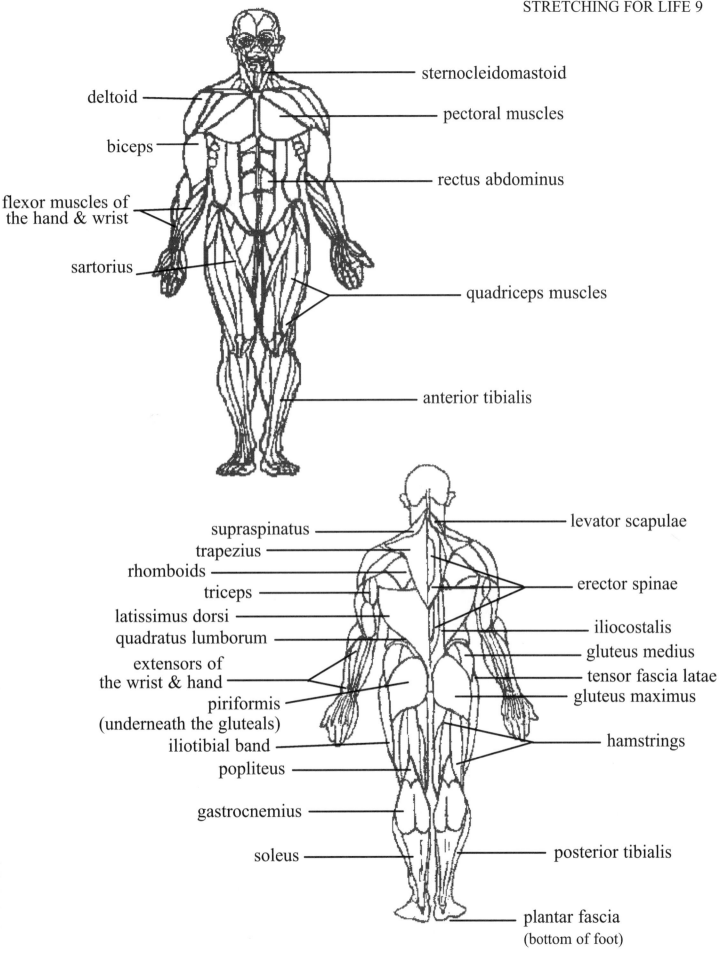

HEAD AND NECK

The muscles of your neck and head serve both to move your head in all directions and to stabilize your head atop your shoulders. These muscles influence the curvature of your spine and affect your posture.

Chronic, postural overload of the neck muscles is due to prolonged, stationary sitting and standing, often with the head tilted forward. This puts a strain on the muscles which extend and rotate the head. Stretching this group of muscles often during the day helps reduce headaches and neckaches.

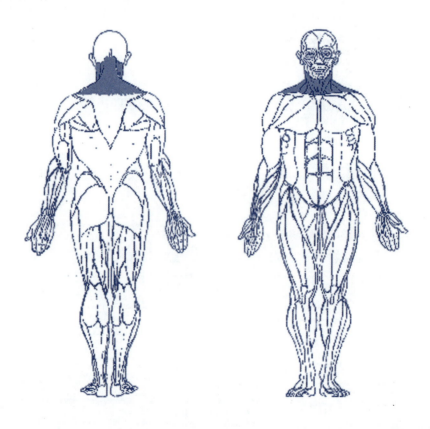

The muscles of the face, jaw and neck will often tighten due to frowning, squinting, clenching of teeth, and from being cold. You can also tighten your neck and shoulder muscles due to emotional upset, temporary trauma, stress, or prolonged inactivity.

There is often a dull, pulling feeling while stretching. If you feel a sharp pain, stop immediately, and check to see if you are doing the stretch correctly. Do it again slowly, and if the pain continues, stop, and try another stretch. If the pain continues, consult a healthcare professional.

STRETCHING FOR LIFE 11

NECK STRETCHES

1 MINUTE NECK RELEASE

Sitting or standing, bend your head to the right, reach your right arm over your head, placing your hand on the left ear. Gently rest the arm on your head, feeling the stretch along the left side of your neck. Hold 20 - 30 seconds. Repeat on the other side. For added stretch, hold onto the chair with your other hand while doing this.

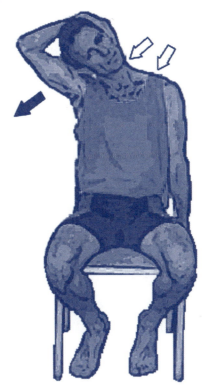

YES-NO-MAYBES

Sitting comfortably, raise your head up and own (nodding your head yes) 5 - 8 times. Turn your head sideways (no) 5 - 8 times. Raise your shoulders up and drop them down (maybe) 5 - 8 times. Do this slowly and easily. This exercise should take you one and a half minutes. Repeat throughout the day. Your neck and shoulders should feel looser afterwards.

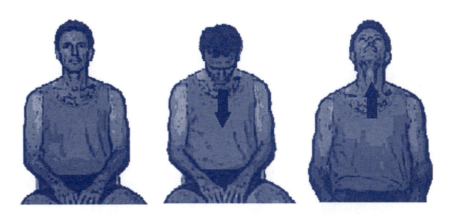

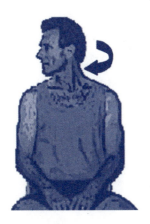 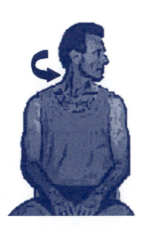 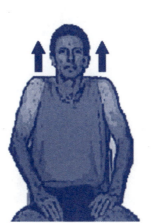 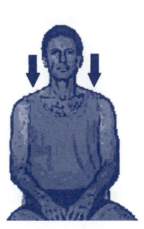

NECK & FACE

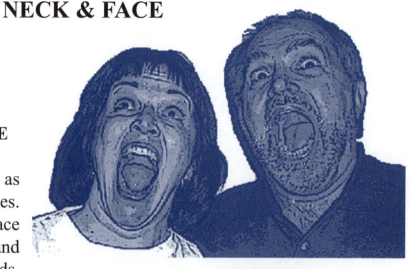

SILENT SCREAM, TINY FACE

Open your eyes and mouth as wide as you can, stretching your face muscles. Hold for 8 seconds. Squeeze your face as tightly as you can with eyes and mouth closed. Hold for 8 seconds. Repeat 3 times. You will feel stretching in a number of places. This takes one minute and can be done anytime, anywhere (when no one is watching). Your face muscles should feel less tense afterwards.

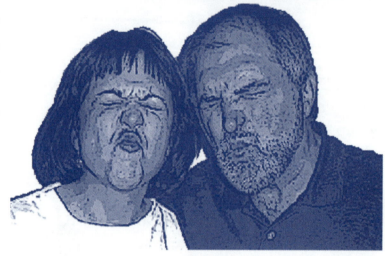

NECK GLIDES
(Turkey Peckers)

Facing a mirror, move your head forward and back in an easy, gliding fashion, keeping your chin and eyes level (don't tilt your head). Move your head forward and back 10 -12 times. Takes about 30 seconds when done slowly. Your neck will feel looser afterwards. You may repeat this stretch 2 - 3 times during the day, or whenever your neck feels tight.

SHOULDERS

How often do you feel like Atlas, the mythical Greek character, carrying the weight of the world on your shoulders? It is quite common to create tightness and soreness in your neck and shoulders, usually from either physical or emotional stress. Long periods of immobility can also create discomfort and restriction in the muscles of your shoulders and upper back.

These stretches will help your upper back and shoulder muscles: rhomboids, trapezius and levator scapulae; the pectoral muscles in the front of the chest; and the shoulder muscles: supraspinatas, deltoid, infraspinatus, subscapularis, teres major and teres minor.

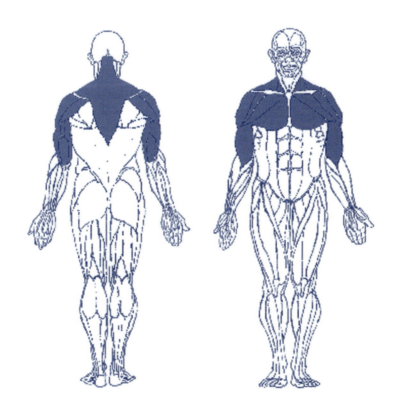

See Appendix, page 49 - "Shouldering Responsibility"
for more information regarding the shoulders.

There is often a dull, pulling feeling while stretching. If you feel a sharp pain, stop immediately, and check to see if you are doing the stretch correctly. Do it again slowly, and if the pain continues, stop, and try another stretch. If the pain continues, consult a healthcare professional.

SHOULDERS/UPPER ARMS

SHOULDER ROLLS
Standing or sitting, lift your shoulders up and forward, then down and back in a rolling motion. Do this easily, keeping your arms and neck relaxed. Do this 10 times, then reverse the direction and roll your shoulders backward 10 times. Takes about one minute to do.

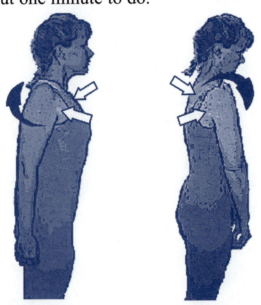

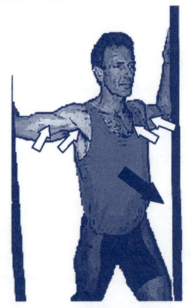

DOORWAY STRETCH
Stand in a doorway and place your arms against the door about shoulder height. Gently lean forward, feeling the stretch in the front of your arms and chest. Hold for 20 - 30 seconds.

DESK SHOULDER STRETCH
Standing with your feet wider than your hips, bend forward at the waist and place your hands on a desk or table. Straighten your arms and allow your back to gently relax. You will feel a stretch in your upper arms, shoulders, and along your back - wherever there is tightness. Breathe. Hold for 20 - 30 seconds.

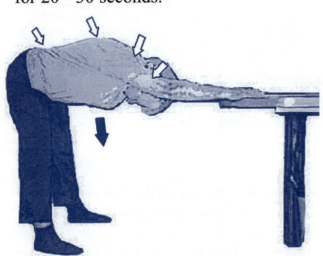

CHEST/SHOULDER STRETCH
Clasp your hands behind your back, and straighten your arms the best you can. You should feel a stretch (almost a burning-like stretch) in your chest and upper arms. As the stretch becomes easier, squeeze your shoulder blades together and lift your arms up to increase the stretch. Hold 20 -30 seconds.

SHOULDERS/UPPER ARMS

TRICEPS STRETCH

Reach over your head and grasp your right elbow. The right hand touches the left shoulder. Slowly pull your arm to the left. You should feel a stretch along the back of the arm. Hold for 20 - 30 seconds, then switch and do the left arm.

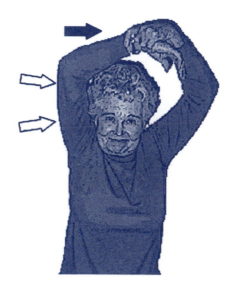

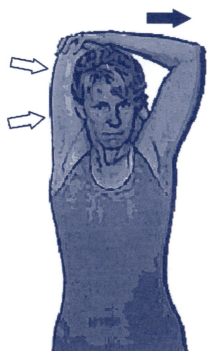

TRICEPS STRETCH (easier)

If you find it difficult to reach over your head to grasp your elbow, try holding your wrist instead. You can still stretch the triceps muscle by pulling your arm over to the other side, holding the stretch for 20 - 30 seconds, then repeat with the other arm.

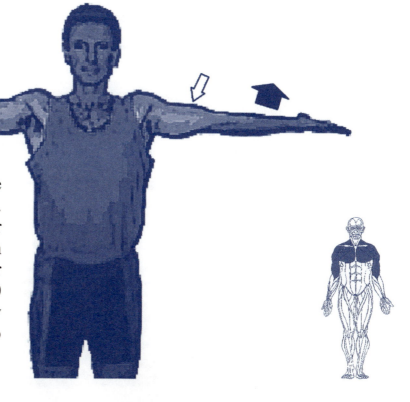

BICEPS STRETCH

Raise your arms out to the side with your palms facing upward. You should feel a stretch in your biceps, which are the muscles in the front of your arm. Relax your shoulders and hold for 20 - 30 seconds. As it gets easier, slowly move your arms backward to increase the stretch.

SHOULDERS/ARMS

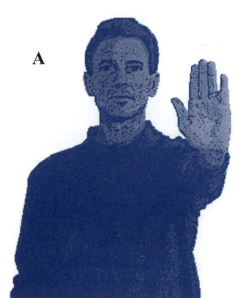

A

THE TRAFFIC COP STRETCH

This is a very effective stretch from the neck down to the wrist. First raise your arm out in front of you with your wrist bent upward (like telling someone to "stop"). Keeping your arm raised, move it out to the side, then turn your head in the opposite direction. You'll feel stretching anywhere from your neck to your shoulder, arm, and wrist. Hold for 20-30 seconds, then repeat on the other side.

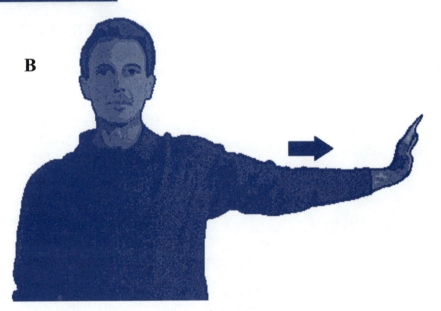

B

C

This stretch may affect any or all of the following muscles: the wrist flexors, biceps, deltoid, scalenes, and sternocleidomastoid. Use it often to prevent a buildup of stress in the neck and wrist, which can lead to neckaches and Carpal Tunnel Syndrome.

ARMS, WRISTS AND HANDS

The muscles of your forearm, wrist and hand have a multitude of responsibilities and movements. Your elbow not only bends and straightens, but also rotates in (pronate) and out (supinate). Your wrist moves up (extension) and down (flexion), side to side (lateral flexion), and in a complete circle (circumduction). Your hand and fingers also open (extend) and close (flex), spread apart (abduction) and come together (adduction).

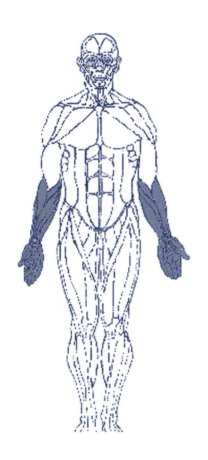

Technically speaking, everyone is taught how to hold and play a musical instrument, with wrists, elbows, and shoulders relaxed. As far as I can tell, no one is taught how to play the computer. It is "here's how you turn it on, and start typing." The problem with that is many people are straining their wrists and tightening their shoulders from improper biomechanics, resulting in common problems such as Carpal Tunnel Syndrome and neckaches. These problems can be prevented with proper wrist and arm alignment, along with daily stretches to alleviate the accumulated tightness that occurs after hours of typing at the keyboard and using the computer mouse.

People also create wrist problems while gardening, sewing, writing, driving and performing small, specific movements. Stretching consistently helps reduce the onset of wrist or hand pain.

See Appendix, page 50, "Cumulative Trauma Disorders"

There is often a dull, pulling feeling while stretching. If you feel a sharp pain, stop immediately, and check to see if you are doing the stretch correctly. Do it again slowly, and if the pain continues, stop, and try another stretch. If the pain continues, consult a healthcare professional.

WRISTS/FOREARMS

STRETCHING YOUR FOREARMS
Place your hands on a desk, table, kitchen counter, or flat surface with your fingers pointing away from you. Gently lean forward. You will feel a stretch along the inside of your arm and wrist. Hold for 20 - 30 seconds. Breathe. Repeat whenever your wrists start to feel tight.

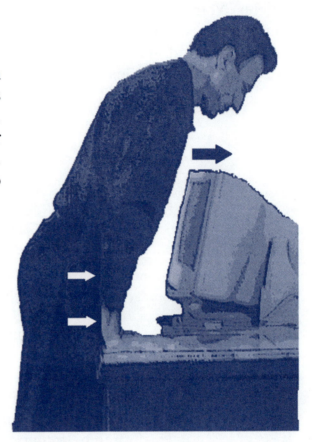

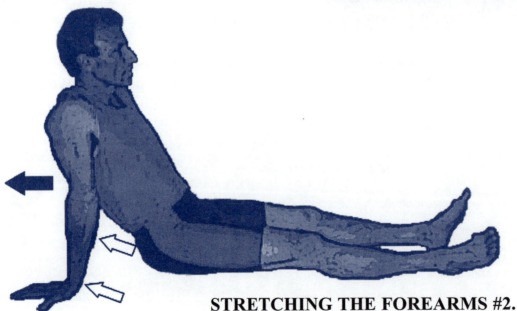

STRETCHING THE FOREARMS #2.
Sit down on the floor, placing your hands on the floor close behind you, fingers pointing away from you. Gently lean backward, feeling the stretch along the inside of your forearm. Hold for 20 - 30 seconds. Breathe.

WRISTS/FOREARMS

WAVES #1
Raise your hands above your head and rotate your wrists around in circles. Rotate them both clockwise and counter-clockwise 15 - 20 seconds in each direction. Your elbows are not moving. Repeat often throughout the day. Your wrists should feel looser after you are finished.

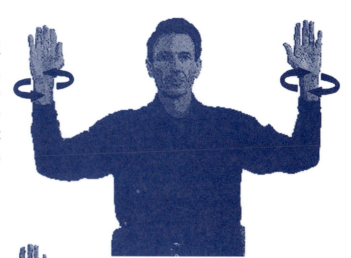

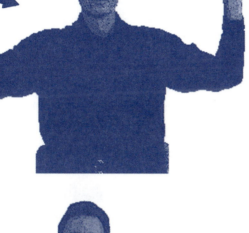

WAVES #2
With your hands above your head, move your wrists side to side for 15 -20 seconds in an easy and gentle manner. Do not move your elbows. You should feel a mild stretch down the sides of your arm, possibly to the elbow. Repeat throughout the day.

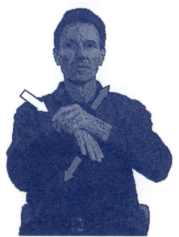 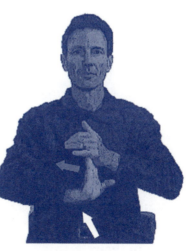

STRETCHING YOUR WRISTS
With your left hand, grab the back of your right hand and gently push down, stretching the back of your hand. Hold for 10 seconds, then push your fingers and hand backwards, stretching the front of your wrist, also for 10 seconds. Repeat 3 times, then switch and do the left hand. You should feel a mild to moderate pulling from the wrist to the forearm. There should be no pain or nerve tingling. If there is, do the wave stretch first (or again), then repeat this stretch. If pain continues, stop, and consult a health care professional.

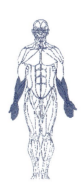

BACK, SPINE & PELVIS

Your spine moves in three directions:
Forward and backward, side to side, and in rotation. It is important that you move your back in all three directions every day. The following stretches give you options for stretching while standing, sitting or lying down. They can be done any time of the day or evening, but they should be done, period. **You will find that stretching your back on a daily basis will often prevent the chronic stiffness and achiness that usually accompanies misuse and disuse of your spine.**

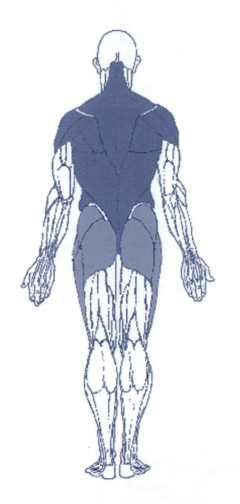

The muscles of your back which affect your posture and overall comfort start with the trapezius muscles at the base of your skull and end at your twelfth rib. You have erector spinae muscles which run the length of your spine from your head to your sacrum (base of your spine). Powerful muscles include the quadratus lumborum muscles which connect your low back to your pelvis and the iliopsoas muscles which attaches on the inside of your spine and connects near the top of your femur (thigh bone). You have small muscles throughout the back which assist in the specific movements of bending and lifting. All these muscles, big and small, can tighten and become painful with inactivity and postural overload.

80% of the adult population in America will suffer from some type of low back pain in their lifetime.

There is often a dull, pulling feeling while stretching. If you feel a sharp pain, stop immediately, and check to see if you are doing the stretch correctly. Do it again slowly, and if the pain continues, stop, and try another stretch. If the pain continues, consult a healthcare professional.

BACK, SPINE & PELVIS

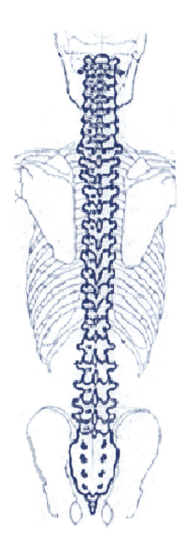

You have 24 moveable vertebrae in your back, held together by nearly 100 muscles, along with ligaments and connective tissue. There are fibrous disks with a spongy center which help hold the vertebrae in place and assist in shock absorption. It is the four curves of the spine, however, which offer you the greatest amount of springiness and shock absorption against the force of gravity.

Your spinal column can be altered over time due to poor posture, trauma and injury, repetitive movement, sports, or improper biomechanics. The misalignment of the vertebrae, along with the muscle imbalance can lead to poor nerve and blood flow, which can lead to inefficient movement, poor performance, and chronic discomfort.

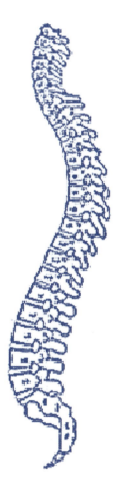

A great portion of our day is spent in flexion; with sitting at a desk, driving a car, and bending forward to work on projects and to pick things up. The muscles which complain the most are the extensors, the muscles which bend us backwards. When they are in a chronic state of flexion, the extensor muscles fatigue and tighten up, causing pain and discomfort. This tightening reveals itself when you lean backward, bend sideways or twist to reach for something behind you.

See Appendix, page 51, "Are You Winning the Battle?"

BACK STRETCHES

TIE CAT/COW

Get on your hands and knees, with your hands directly under your shoulders, and knees directly under your hips. Arch your back up, tuck your pelvis under, and drop your chin to your chest. Hold for 4 seconds, then drop your back down, push your pelvis back and lift your head. Hold for 4 seconds. Your elbows stay straight and do not bend. Repeat 6 - 8 times. Do this slowly and easily. It is easiest to breathe in going down and exhaling going up.

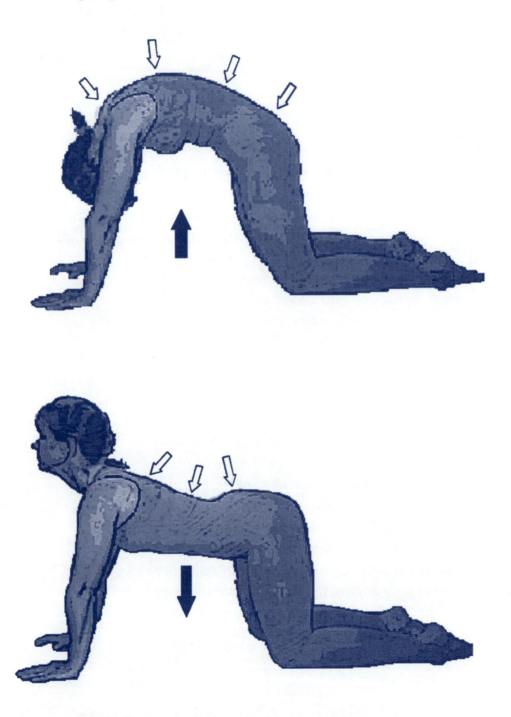

EXTENSION STRETCHES

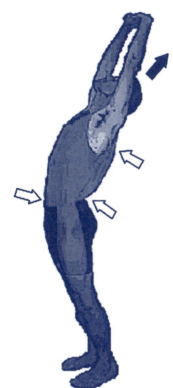
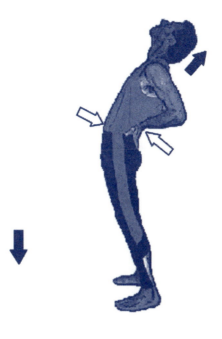
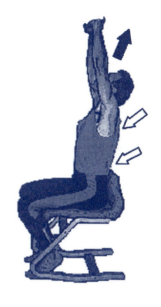

EXTENSION #1
Standing, clasp your hands together over your head and gently lean backwards for 10 seconds. You should feel a stretch in your low back, in the back of your shoulders, and in the front of your hips. Relax, then repeat 1 - 2 more times.

EXTENSION #2 (easier)
Should you find it difficult to lift both arms above your head as shown in version #1, place your hands on your low back, then lean backwards and do the stretch. You'll feel a stretch in your low back and in the front of your hips. Hold for 10 seconds, relax, then repeat 1 - 2 more times.

SEATED EXTENSIONS
(for those who don't want to get up)
Grasp your hands above your head, sit up and lean backwards. You should feel the stretch in your low back, upper arms, and neck. Hold for 10 - 30 seconds, then relax and repeat 1 - 2 more times. Breathe slowly and easily.

THE SPHINX
When stretching on the floor, lie on your stomach and elbows. Lift your head and upper body off the floor (A) and feel a stretch in both the low back and the hip flexors. Hold for 10 - 15 seconds. Relax and take a breath. Lift up again, either on your elbows or pushing yourself up higher with your hands on the floor, arms straight (B). Hold for 10 -15 seconds. Breathe.

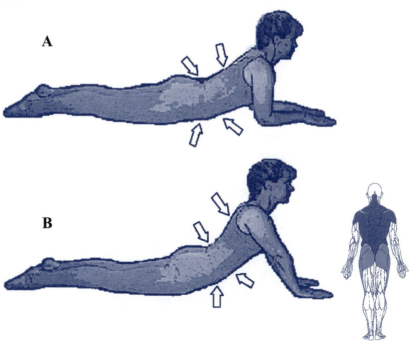

FLEXION STRETCHES

FLEXION #1
Lying on you back, bend your knees and gently pull them towards your chest. Hold for 10 seconds, relax for one breath, then gently pull your knees closer to your chest. Repeat 2 - 3 more times, holding for at least 10 seconds each time. Breathe easily.

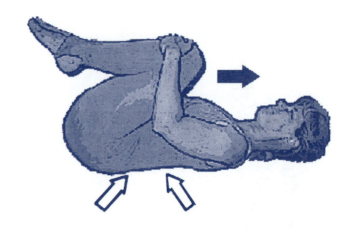

FLEXION #2
Another great stretch, very effective for the low back, hips and buttocks, is sitting crosslegged on the floor. Sit up straight, then slowly lean forward over your legs. You'll feel the stretch all along your back. Attempt to place your hands onto the floor. Hold for 30 - 60 seconds. Breathe.

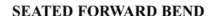

SEATED FORWARD BEND
Sit in a chair, knees apart, and lean forward with your hands touching the floor. Relax your head, shoulders and arms. You should feel the stretch along your spine. Hold for 30 - 60 seconds. Remember to breathe.

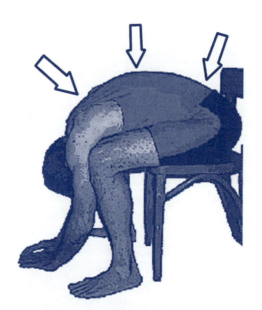

THE PLOW (ADVANCED)
Some people can do this stretch easily. Lie on your back and bring your legs up over your head, keeping them as straight as possible. Your weight is on your shoulders, not your neck. Let the weight of your legs help in stretching your back. Breathe. Hold for 30 - 60 seconds.

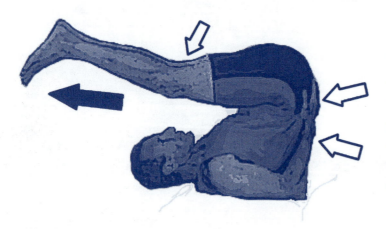

ROTATION STRETCHES

TRUNK ROTATION - LYING DOWN

Lying on your back, bend your knees and drop your legs to the right, resting the right leg on the floor. Keep your left shoulder and arm on the floor and turn your head to the left side. Breathe. Hold this position for 1 minute. You will feel the stretch mostly along the left side of your back. Lift your knees and drop them to the floor on the left side and hold 1 minute. You will feel your back muscles relax the longer you hold the stretch.

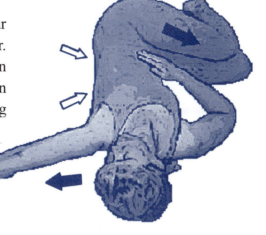

SEATED TWIST

Sitting in a chair, sit up straight and twist behind you, looking over your shoulder. Grab the back of the chair with your arm and gently push yourself further into the stretch. Breathe. Hold for 10 - 20 seconds, then repeat on the other side. Repeat this 2 times. The second time should be easier.

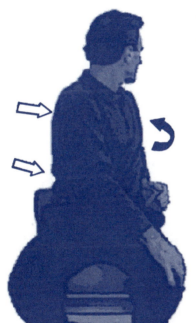

STANDING TWIST

Stand facing a wall or doorway. With your left hand, reach across to the right and place your hand on the wall. Push against the wall as you twist to the right, looking over your right shoulder. You'll feel a stretching the right side of your back from the waist to your shoulder blade. Hold for 20 - 30 seconds, then turn and repeat on the left side. Repeat this 2 times. The second time should be easier. Remember to breathe.

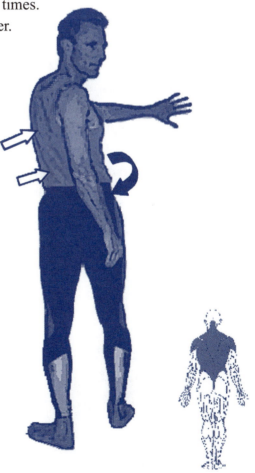

LATERAL SIDE STRETCHES

Stretching side to side allows for lengthening of the paraspinal muscles, low back muscles, and the muscles of your shoulder and upper back. The best way to side stretch is standing, feet spread wider than your hips. Right hand rests on the knee or thigh and the left arm is raised over your head. Reach up and over, but do not "collapse" at the waist or bend forward. Hold for 20 - 30 seconds, then repeat on the other side. You will feel the stretch in your back and along the left hip, ribs and the neck.

SIDE STRETCH # 2 (easier)
If you have difficulty raising either arm above your head, due to an injury or shoulder restriction, you can still stretch to the side. Place your left hand on a wall, arm straight. Cross your left leg over the right, then lean towards the wall, stretching your left side. Hold for 20 - 30 seconds, then repeat on the right side. You will feel the stretch along the left hip, ribs and in your back.

SEATED SIDEBEND
Sitting upright in a chair, raise your left arm up over your head and lean to the right. You should feel the stretch along the left side of your back, neck and ribs and under your left shoulder. Make sure your neck and head are relaxed. Hold for 20 - 30 seconds, then repeat on the other side. Remember to breathe.

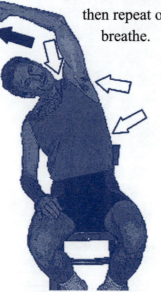

SEATED SIDEBEND (easier)
If you have trouble lifting either arm above your head, you can still do a side stretch. Sit up straight, then lean to the right, allowing your right arm to hang down and your left shoulder to roll forward, adding extra "stretch". Relax your neck and head. Hold for 20 - 30 seconds, then repeat on the other side.

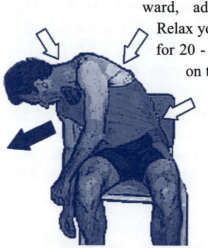

HIPS/PELVIS

SEATED CROSS-LEGGED STRETCH

Sit up straight in your chair, crossing the right ankle on to the left knee. Slowly lean forward, keeping your back as straight as possible. You should feel a stretch in the right hip/buttock/thigh. Hold for 20 - 30 seconds, then repeat with the left leg. Remember to breathe.

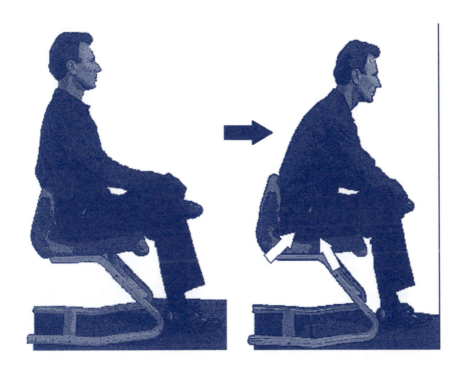

HIP/PIRIFORMIS STRETCH

This stretch is easier than it looks. Lie down on your back, cross your left ankle onto your right knee. Reach in and grab the back of your right leg and pull. This will create a stretch in the left buttock muscles. If you straighten the right leg, you will get a small stretch in the back of the knee. Hold for 20 - 30 seconds, then repeat with the right leg. It doesn't matter whether your head is resting on the floor or off the floor.

HIPS/PELVIS

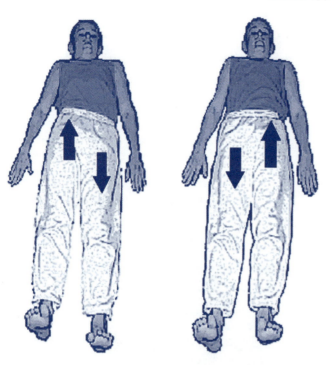

HIP RAISES

Lying on your back, either in bed or on the floor, raise up the right hip (toward your shoulder, not the ceiling) and push the left hip down. Your legs stay flat on the bed. Then switch and raise the left hip and push down the right. Slowly alternate sides 8 to 12 times. This is a rocking motion with each hip alternating high and low. You will feel stretching anywhere in your low back, hips, groin or buttocks.

PELVIC ROCKS

Lie on your back, either in bed or on the floor. Slowly rock the front of your pelvis upward, pressing your low back into the bed or floor (A). Then slowly rock the front of your pelvis downward, lifting your low back off the bed (B). Repeat this motion for 30 - 60 seconds, in a relaxed fashion. Breathe easily. You should feel stretching in the low back, the groin, and hips.

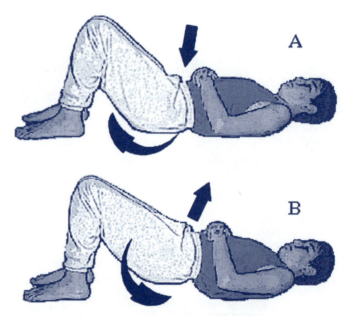

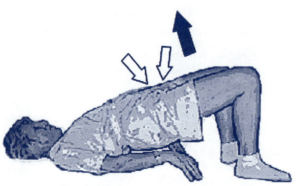

PELVIC BRIDGES

Lying on your back, arms at your side, lift your pelvis up off the floor. Hold this position for 20 - 30 seconds. You should feel tightening in your thighs and buttocks and stretching in the front of your hips (hip flexor muscles). Breathe, and relax your shoulders, arms and feet.

LEGS/FEET

Prolonged sitting or standing, without taking a break, can cause dis-ease in the legs, pelvis or low back. Daily inactivity, with very little movement will lead to shortening of the hip flexors and quadriceps muscles in the front of the thigh. This can then cause tightness and discomfort in the low back, buttocks and hamstrings (back of thigh). You can also alter your balance due to temporary traumas to the ankles, knees or hips. This creates restriction and tightness in your knee or ankle and will often create uneven posture, stiff joints, achy muscles, and restricted range of motion in the back or on the opposite side from the trauma (a sprained left ankle can cause achiness or discomfort in the right knee or hip).

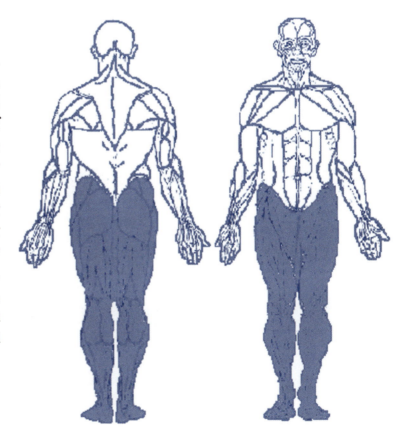

The way you stand, the surfaces you stand on, the shoes you wear, and how long a period of time you spend standing greatly affects the health of your feet and legs. Wearing high heels creates a greater load on your calves, knees and thighs, which can lead to fatigue and cramping in your legs. Standing on hard surfaces for long periods of time will not only fatigue your legs, but also your back. Wearing shoes with good support, taking breaks, and stretching often helps reduce potential discomfort in your legs and back.

See Appendix, page 52, "The not so Psilent Psoas"

There is often a dull, pulling feeling while stretching. If you feel a sharp pain, stop immediately, and check to see if you are doing the stretch correctly. Do it again slowly, and if the pain continues, stop, and try another stretch. If the pain continues, consult a healthcare professional.

QUADRICEPS/HIP FLEXORS

HIP FLEXORS/FRONT OF THIGH
This is an important stretch for anyone who sits a lot. Place your left foot out in front of you, bending the knee no more than 90 degrees. Place the right leg behind you as far as you can, and slowly lean forward, stretching the front of the right thigh. Hold for 20 - 30 seconds. Repeat with the left leg. The heel of the right leg is off the ground.

QUADRICEPS: # 1
The easiest way to stretch the front of your thigh is to bend your knee and grasp your ankle, gently pulling your leg back until you feel a stretch along the front of your thigh. Hold for 20 - 30 seconds, then repeat with the other leg.

VARIATION
To increase the stretch, raise the arm on the same side of the leg you are stretching.

QUADRICEPS: # 2 (easier)
If you find it difficult to bend your knee and grasp your ankle, modify the stretch by placing your bent leg onto a chair. Slowly lean backward until you feel the stretch in the front of your thigh. Hold for 20 - 30 seconds, then repeat with the other leg.

FLOOR QUADRICEPS STRETCH
Lie down on your left side, head resting on your arm or a pillow. Reach back and grasp your right ankle with your right hand and slowly pull your leg backwards. You should feel a stretch along the front of the thigh. Hold for 20 - 30 seconds. Breathe. Relax, switch sides and repeat the stretch.

HAMSTRINGS (back of your thighs)

HAMSTRING STRETCH - LYING DOWN
Lie on the floor, legs straight. Bring one leg up and grasp it behind the knee or thigh. Slowly pull your leg back straightening the leg as much as you can. You should feel the stretch along the back of your thigh. Relax your neck and shoulders. Hold for 20 - 30 seconds. Repeat with the other leg.

SITTING HAMSTRING STRETCH
Sitting on the floor, stretch one leg in front of you, bending the other leg inward. Sit up straight, then lean forward towards the stretched leg reaching for your ankle, toes or bottom of your foot. You should feel a stretch along the back of your thigh. Hold for 20 - 30 seconds. Breathe and relax into the stretch. Repeat with the other leg.

STANDING HAMSTRING STRETCH
Standing next to a chair, sofa back, counter, or wall, place your heel onto the surface and stand up straight. Leaning forward, reach to grab your ankle, toes or the bottom of your foot. You'll feel the stretch along the back of your leg. Breathe and slowly attempt to move your chest to your knee. Hold for 20 - 30 seconds. Repeat with the other leg.

BENDING HAMSTRING STRETCH
Bend forward, placing your chest on your right knee and your left leg behind you. Slowly begin straightening your right leg. keeping your chest as close to your knee as possible. You'll feel the stretch along the back of your thigh. Breathe. Hold for 20 - 30 seconds. Repeat with the other leg.

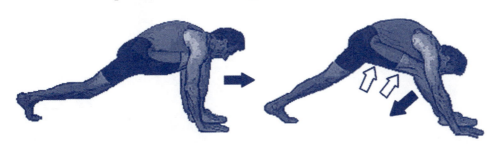
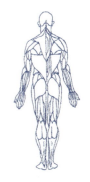

CALF & ANKLE STRETCHES

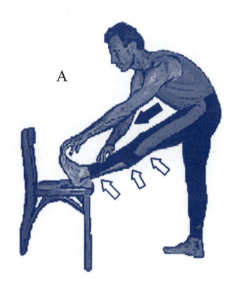

BENDING CALF STRETCH

Standing on the right leg, place your left foot on a chair or low table (A), or keep it on the ground (B). Keeping your back as straight as possible, reach over and grab the left foot/toes. Gently pull up on the foot, stretching the back of your leg. You should feel a stretch in the calf from your heel to the back of your knee. Hold for 20 - 30 seconds. Breathe. Repeat with the right leg.

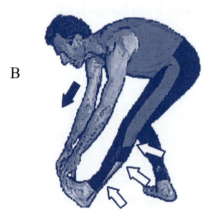

STANDING CALF STRETCH

Place your hands on a wall and put one leg in front and the other behind you. The back foot is standing on a rolled up towel. This helps prevent your arch from flattening and decreasing the effectiveness of the stretch. Bend the front knee and push the heel of your back foot into the floor. You should feel a stretch along the back of your calf from the heel to the back of your knee. Hold for 20 - 30 seconds, then switch legs.

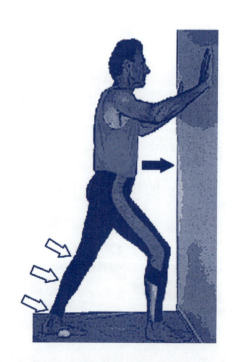

CALF & ANKLE STRETCHES

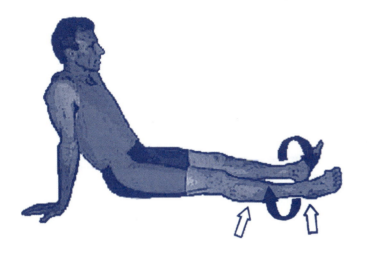

ANKLE ROTATIONS
Either lying or sitting in bed or on the floor, rotate your ankles clockwise 10 - 12 times, then reverse and rotate them counterclockwise the same amount. You should feel a stretch in your calves and in the ankles

SQUATTING CALF/FOOT STRETCH
This is a simple and gentle way to stretch out your calves and the bottom of your feet (if you can kneel on the floor without any knee problems). Kneel on the floor with your toes, knees and hands on the floor. Lift your knees off the floor and gently push backward, increasing the stretch on your calves and the bottom of your feet. Rock easily back and forth, relaxing and stretching the muscles for 20 - 30 seconds. Should you experience any problems, try doing this one leg at a time.

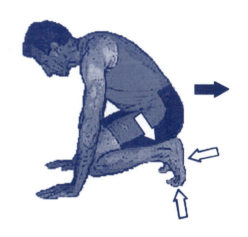

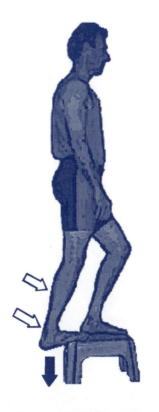

STEP STRETCH
Standing on a step, place the heel of the right foot over the edge of the step. Slowly drop your heel below the level of the step, feeling a stretch in the calf from your heel to the back of your knee. Hold for 20 - 30 seconds. Repeat with the left leg.

STRETCHING ROUTINES - 4 MINUTES OR LESS

Now that you have learned the stretches, you will find that combining the stretches for different situations will help reduce built-up stress and tension. Also, stretching for a few minutes helps lengthen tight muscles that have been inactive for hours at a time. Therefore, the routines are grouped together for the maximum amount of stretching in a minimal amount of time.

Most stretches can also be done by themselves. If your neck feels tight or your arms are sore from working on a project, stopping to take a break and stretching the muscles with even one stretch will help reduce accumulated tightness.

As always, gently do each stretch without bouncing or any forceful action. Make sure your muscles are warmed up whenever possible. Start the stretch slowly, and once you reach what feels like the end of the stretch, breath, and allow the muscles to relax. The pulling, stretchy feeling should fade as you continue the stretch, and it is normal for the muscle to feel warmer after the stretch is finished.

Use the stretches that best suit your body type and your lifestyle. You should make up your own 4 - minute stretching routines. This will help you stretch more often during the day.

REMINDER: Black arrows ➡ tell you which way to move,

White arrows ⇨ tell you where you should feel the stretch

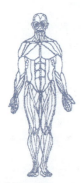

STRETCHING FOR LIFE 35

WAKE UP STRETCHES — 2-3 minutes

Feel stiff in the morning? Some stiffness in the joints upon waking is normal. This is due to the fact that you have been lying horizontal for 6 to 8 hours, and the "extra" cellular fluid in your body has ended up in the joints. Moving around helps relieve this stress as your body's fluids transfer into other areas.

Before you get out of bed, gently wake up your muscles by doing the following routine.

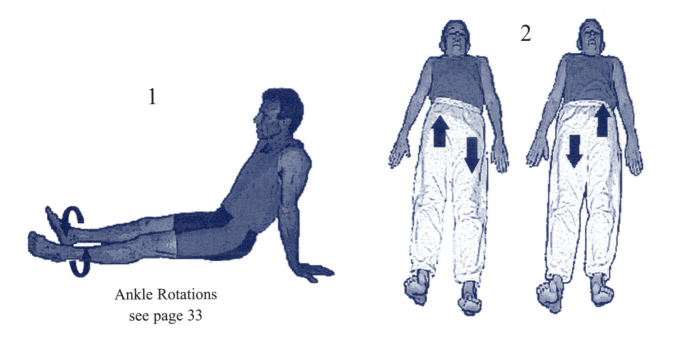

Ankle Rotations
see page 33

Hip Raises - 8 to 12 times
see page 28

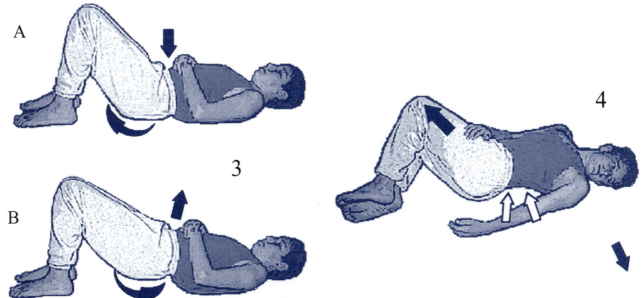

Pelvic Rocks - 30 to 60 seconds
see page 28

Trunk Rotation - 30 to 60 seconds
see page 25

BACK ROUTINE #1 — 4 minutes

These three stretches address all ranges of motion for the back, and they, or similar stretches, should be done everyday, for the rest of your life.

CAT COW - 8 to 10 times
see page 22

Trunk Rotation
30 to 60 seconds each side
see page 25

Lateral Side Bends
30 seconds each side
see page 26

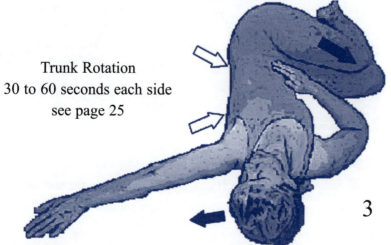

STRETCHING FOR LIFE 37

BACK ROUTINE #2 — (seated) 4 minutes

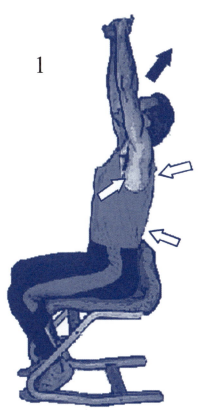

Extension 30 seconds
see page 23

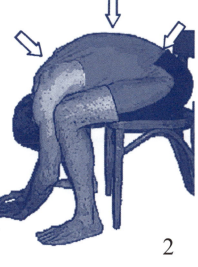

Flexion
30 seconds
see page 24

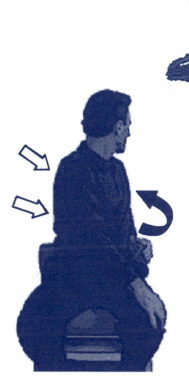

Rotation
30 seconds each side
see page 25

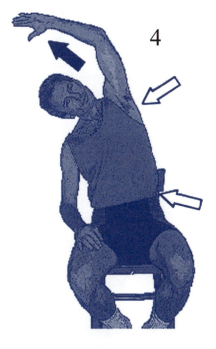

Lateral Side Bends
30 seconds each side
see page 26

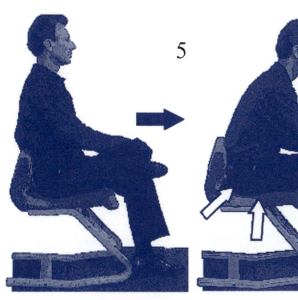

Seated Cross-legged stretch
30 seconds each side
see page 27

BACK STRETCHES # 3 — (Floor) 3-1/2 Minutes

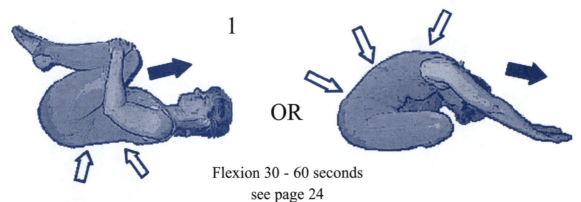

1

Flexion 30 - 60 seconds
see page 24

2

a

b

Pelvic Rocks
lift 10 to 12 times - 60 seconds
see page 25

3

Hip/Piriformis Stretch
30 seconds each leg
see page 27

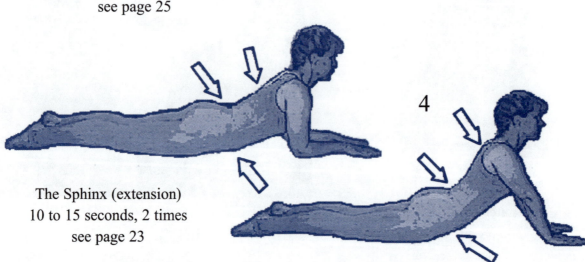

4

The Sphinx (extension)
10 to 15 seconds, 2 times
see page 23

STRETCHING FOR LIFE 39

NECK & FACE — 4 Minutes

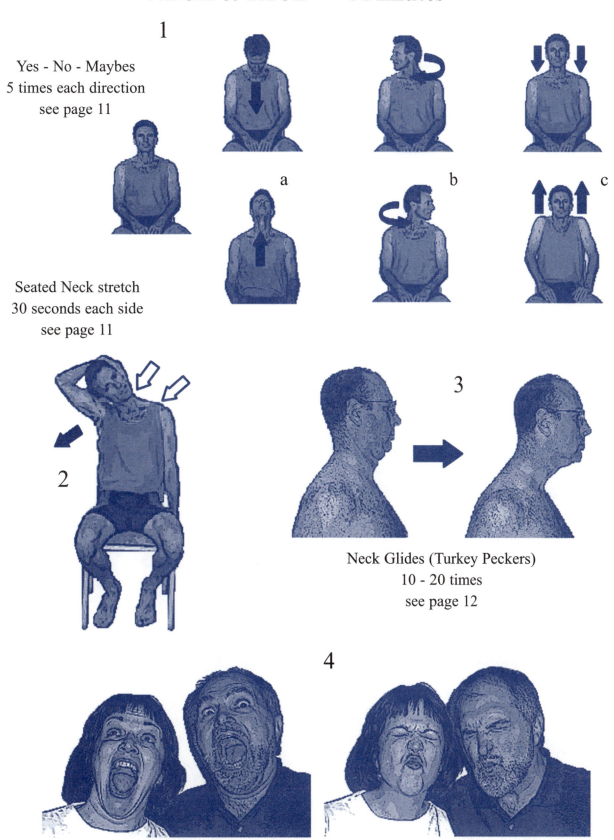

Yes - No - Maybes
5 times each direction
see page 11

Seated Neck stretch
30 seconds each side
see page 11

Neck Glides (Turkey Peckers)
10 - 20 times
see page 12

Silent Scream, Tiny Face
8 seconds wide, 8 seconds closed, repeat 3 times
see page 12

OFFICE #1 — 4 Minutes

Studies have shown that workers who take hourly breaks from their tasks remain more alert and have greater productivity than those workers who take few to no breaks during the day.

1

EXTENSION
30 seconds
see page 23

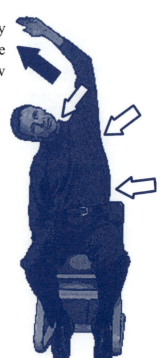

2

SIDEBENDS
30 seconds each side
see page 26

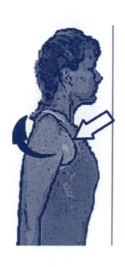

3

SHOULDER ROLLS
30 seconds
see page 14

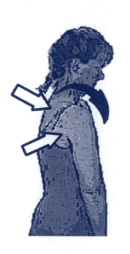

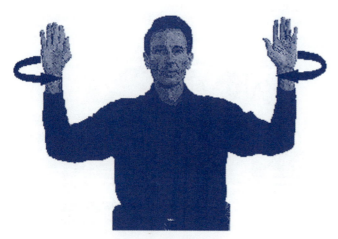

4 WAVES
30 seconds
see page 19

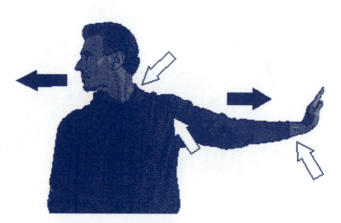

TRAFFIC COP STRETCH **5**
30 seconds each side
see page 16

STRETCHING FOR LIFE 41

OFFICE #2 — (standing)

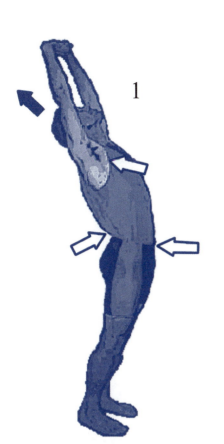

EXTENSION
30 seconds
see page 23

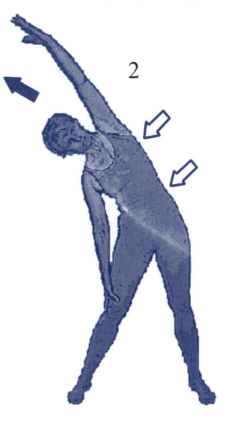

SIDEBENDS
30 seconds each side
see page 26

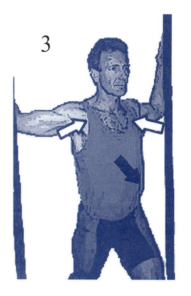

DOORWAY STRETCH
30 seconds
see page 14

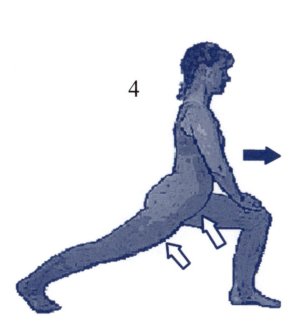

The LUNGE
30 seconds each leg
see page 30

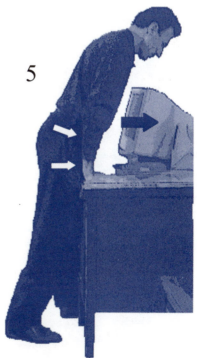

STANDING WRIST STRETCH
30 seconds
see page 18

TRAVELING — (sitting) 4 minutes

When you are traveling by car or airplane, you are often confined to your seat for long periods of time, and if you are squeezed in next to someone, you don't always have a lot of room to move. These four stretches allow you to stretch with the least amount of movement.

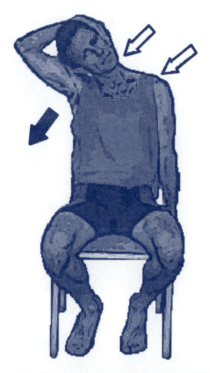

1 MINUTE NECK STRETCH
30 seconds each side
see page 11

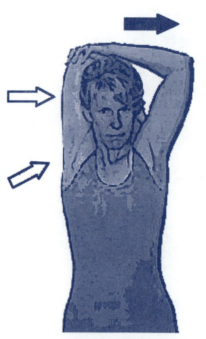

TRICEPS STRETCH
30 seconds each side
see page 15

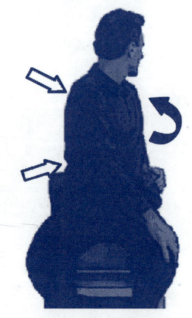

SEATED TWIST
30 seconds each side
see page 25

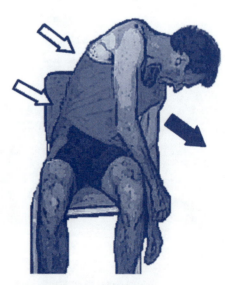

SEATED SIDEBEND
30 seconds each side
see page 26

STRETCHING FOR LIFE 43

TRAVELING — (standing) 4 minutes

At the first opportunity to stop when traveling, stand up and move your muscles. Stiff joints and tight muscles occur with prolonged inactivity, and stretching helps relax them. It also helps to walk and move around for a few minutes before returning to your seat or getting back into the car.

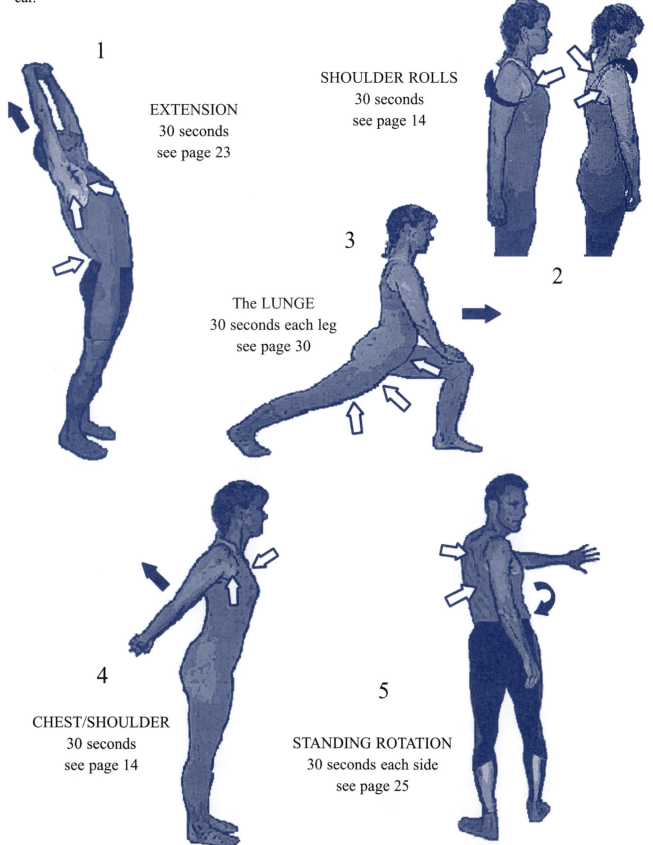

1. EXTENSION
30 seconds
see page 23

2. SHOULDER ROLLS
30 seconds
see page 14

3. The LUNGE
30 seconds each leg
see page 30

4. CHEST/SHOULDER
30 seconds
see page 14

5. STANDING ROTATION
30 seconds each side
see page 25

WARM-UP Lower Body #1 — 3 to 3-1/2 minutes

Use these stretches prior to walking/jogging, bicycling, skiing, racquet sports, and others.

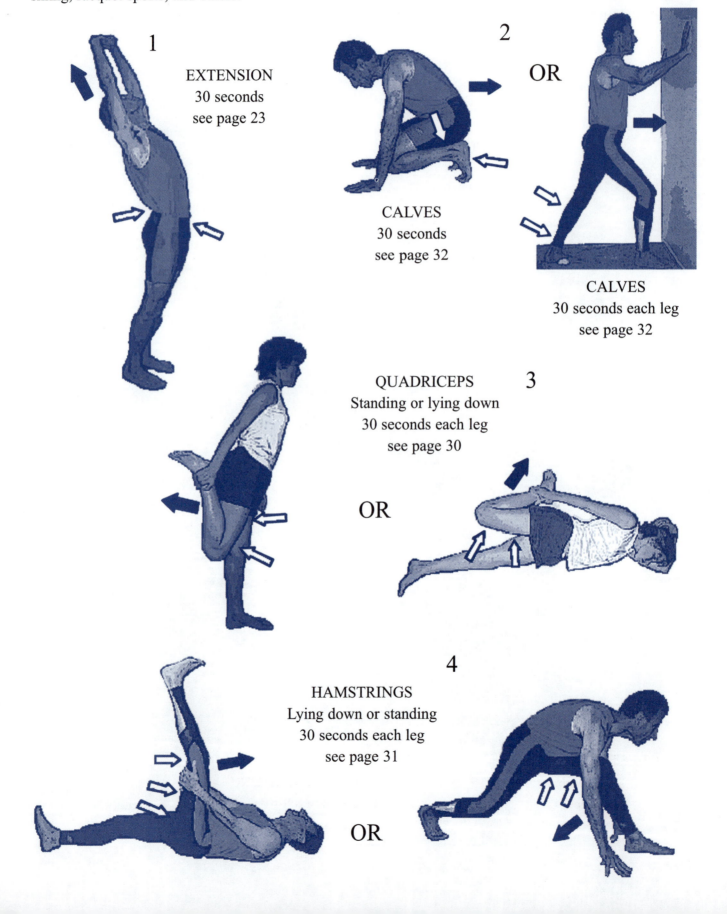

1 EXTENSION
30 seconds
see page 23

2 CALVES
30 seconds
see page 32

OR

CALVES
30 seconds each leg
see page 32

3 QUADRICEPS
Standing or lying down
30 seconds each leg
see page 30

OR

4 HAMSTRINGS
Lying down or standing
30 seconds each leg
see page 31

OR

WARM UP - Lower Body #2 — 4 minutes

These stretches are good for your legs prior to any sport, game or activity.

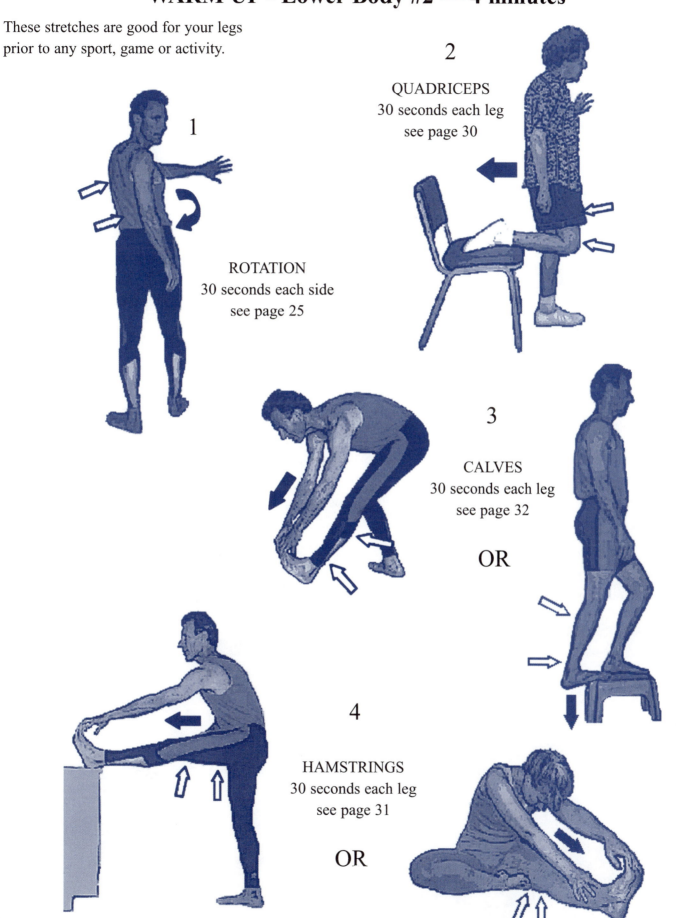

1 ROTATION
30 seconds each side
see page 25

2 QUADRICEPS
30 seconds each leg
see page 30

3 CALVES
30 seconds each leg
see page 32
OR

4 HAMSTRINGS
30 seconds each leg
see page 31
OR

STRETCHING FOR LIFE 45

46

WARM-UP Upper Body — 4 minutes

Use the following routine to stretch the arms and upper body prior to activities or sports such as gardening, baseball, softball, volleyball, basketball, frisbee, etc.

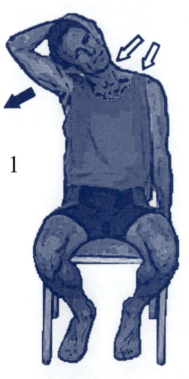

1

1 MINUTE NECK RELEASE
30 seconds each side
see page 11
(can do standing or sitting)

2

CHEST/SHOULDER
30 seconds
see page 14

3

TRICEPS
30 seconds each side
see page 15

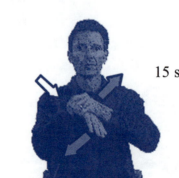

WRISTS
15 seconds each direction
both hands
see page 19

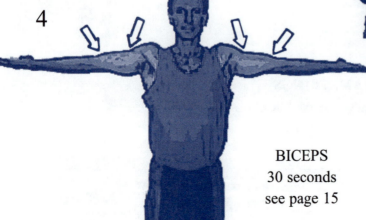

4

BICEPS
30 seconds
see page 15

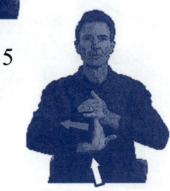

5

APPENDIX

Most of the following articles are from my newsletter <u>Body Briefs</u>, a bi-monthly publication I began writing in 1993. They are here to provide you with further information regarding stretching, posture, injuries, and muscle function. Additional articles maybe found on my website, ***www.stretching4life.com***.

Efficient Posture 48

Shouldering Responsibility 49

Cumulative Trauma Disorders 50

Are You Winning the Battle? 51

The Not-So-Psilent Psoas 52

Power Stance 53

Slouching Towards Retirements 54

EFFICIENT POSTURE:

Sitting and working at a desk for prolonged periods of time tends to tighten and stiffen your muscles, particularly the neck, shoulders, back, wrist, and hands. Maintaining a balanced and efficient posture helps reduce the build-up of tension and muscular shortening.

Head should be resting over the shoulders in a neutral position.

The top of the computer screen should be at or near eye level.

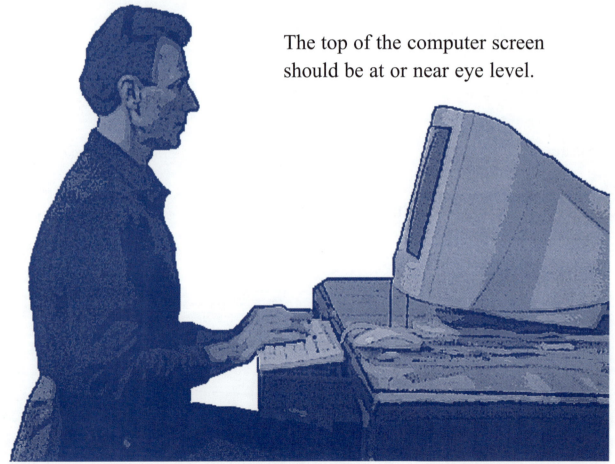

Elbows should be bent close to 90°.
Wrists should be in a relaxed and neutral position, hardly bent at all.

SHOULDERING RESPONSIBILITY

Do you ever have periods of time when things repeat themselves? You hear the word efficacious said by three different people in the same day or you see five red Mustang convertibles in a week. Well, for me, this was "shoulder" month. It just seemed like a lot of people came in with shoulder problems, so I would like to explain to you how and why your shoulder works the way it does.

The shoulder is a **ball and socket** joint. While this allows for great *mobility*, it creates a decrease in *stability*. The humerus (upper arm bone) is the ball" which fits into a "socket" created by your scapula (shoulder blade) and your clavicle (collar bone). This joint is held together by ligaments and a number of muscles, including a group called the **rotator cuff** muscles. These muscles enable you to move your arm forward and backward, rotate inward and outward, away from and toward your body, and swing the arm in a full circle.

The make-up of the shoulder joint, like all the other joints in the body, consists of a joint capsule surrounded by ligaments (bone to bone), tendons (muscle to bone), fascia (connective tissue), bursa (cellular padding), and a network of nerves called the brachial plexus. Any one of these components can malfunction and result in pain and dysfunction.

When there is a trauma to the shoulder region, such as a dislocation or separation, a pattern of pain dysfunction and rehabilitation is fairly predictable. When there is *sustained* injury, due to repetitive stress, chronic overload and fatigue, or poor biomechanics in work or play, then there is the potential for tendinitis, bursitis, capsulitis or myofascitis. Any of these inflammatory conditions can cause pain, loss of strength or decrease in range of motion.

Chiropractic care can often help with these types of conditions because most of the muscles in the shoulder region attach themselves to the *axial* skeleton, which is the spine and ribs. By determining the underlying cause of the problem we increase the opportunity for creating the right environment for healing.

One of the most common and preventable causes of pain in the shoulder is poor biomechanics. Poor posture due to improper chair or desk height, slouching in a sofa or chair, or holding the steering wheel in a "death grip". All these postures can contribute to fatigue and musculoskeletal imbalance, which in turn can lead to pain while engaged in other activities. When you can learn to relax your shoulders when under stress, and change the way you sit, type, drive or write, then the healing process will begin and the chronic problem eliminated.

Remember, it's not humerus to have shoulder pain.

BODY BRIEFS, September, 1994

CUMULATIVE TRAUMA DISORDERS
and how to prevent them

Cumulative trauma disorders (CTDs) are conditions caused by the continuous and repetitive use of muscles, tendons, ligaments, joints and nerves. They can occur in nearly every area of the body, but the most common areas are the wrist and low back. The symptoms of tightness, stiffness, numbness, pain or discomfort, tingling or loss of strength and stability are due to an inflammatory breakdown of that particular body part. CTDs will develop over long periods of time and are chronic in nature. This is why it is necessary to get up and move often throughout the day and to incorporate a regular stretching program which will relax and release accumulated stress and tension.

Common causes can occur from over-activities involving constant repetitiveness, lifting heavy loads or improper body mechanics. How you sit, stand, grip, lift, carry, type, sew, repair, pull, push, assemble, or play a sport has an inherent risk of injury, particularly if there are faulty body mechanics and or the absence of adequate rest.

Because stretching affects the muscles, tendons and joints, the first line of defense against CTDs is to stretch daily to prevent, or at least reduce, the risk of creating a CTD somewhere. This stretching should be coupled with adequate rest in order for the body to repair itself and recover from prolonged activity.

Another line of defense against CTDs is good posture. This comes from an awareness of your body position, how long you stay immobile, and how much excess stress is influencing your activity. Often simple adjustments in chair or desk height or repositioning equipment to a more accessible place helps in eliminating potential problems.

While some occupations have a greater risk of creating CTDs, and some body types tend to have a greater risk of incurring CTDs, all CTDs are preventable at some point in time. If you start performing a new activity incorrectly, then the chance of preventing a problem in the future is diminished. If you work, or play, so hard and for so long that you never allow yourself time to rest, then the odds of you creating a CTD increase dramatically. Remember, you were not born with back pain or Carpal Tunnel Syndrome, and many people never get a CTD in their life, so why should you?

ARE YOU WINNING THE BATTLE?

What battle? You didn't even know there was a war. Actually, it's your battle with gravity, and it's either for you or against you. Gravity is constantly challenging you: as I pull you down, what are you going to do? How are you going to keep yourself upright?

Relating to these questions, I read an interesting article recently on <u>Muscular Intelligence</u> by Cam Cameron, who stated some very interesting observations regarding gravity and your posture. First, "gravity never takes a day off". Secondly, "the human body is an adaptable machine, which will (positively) condition itself to intelligent demand or (negatively) de-condition itself with unthinking habitual repetition."

If gravity is constantly pulling you down, shouldn't you respond by springing upward? If you do not have upward spring then you compress your body and slump (or slouch). Your ligaments, cartilage and discs all suffer a breakdown in muscular or postural intelligence, and all for the sake of comfort or the "path of least resistance."

Slumping is the unconscious sabotaging of your skeletal design, which can lead to negative compensations throughout the body. Compressed hips and sacroiliac joints can lead to low back stiffness and weakness. Thoracic spine collapse compresses the rib cage - smaller breaths - and forces the head forward, putting greater pressure on the base of the neck and base of the head. This can create headaches, neck pain, and tight shoulders and neck.

By shifting your posture into an "S" curve (S is for springing), you lift your chest up, relaxing the shoulder muscles and bringing the head back to rest on the shoulders. The pelvis is more level, allowing back muscles to relax and an expanded rib cage to breathe easier.

So, when you are standing or sitting, observe whether you are in an "S" posture (springing up) or in a "C" curve (collapsing), and adjust your body accordingly. Then you can smile and say to gravity, "See, I'm winning. Ha!"

BODY BRIEFS, September, 2000

THE NOT-SO-PSILENT PSOAS

There is a muscle deep inside your back which is the main force that helps you bend forward or lift your leg, known as the iliopsoas (ileo-soaz) muscle. The function of this muscle is *hip flexion, lateral rotation* and *abduction* (lifting your leg away from your body). It is often involved in acute low back and sciatic cases, along with postural distortions such as scoliosis and sway back (hyperlordosis).

The psoas is a powerful muscle that is attached to the inside of your low back (L1 to L5 vertebrae), travels across your pelvis and attaches to the inside of your femur (thigh bone). When there is tension in the psoas, the pain can mimic kidney or gall bladder disease. Often, it is involved in that deep, aching pain in your low back.

The psoas does not stand alone, however. Its involvement is usually associated with spasm of the lower back muscles and tightness in the abdominal muscles. It is often difficult to relax the lower back muscles without also releasing the psoas. When one psoas muscle is in spasm, you often see a forward and sideways tilt in a person's posture. When both psoas muscles are spasmed, the tendency is to lean forward to help ease the pain.

The most common situations which can inflame or spasm the psoas are those where an excess load is placed on the low back while lifting. Reaching in to lift something out of the trunk of your car and then twisting with the load can potentially overload the low back and cause a major back problem. Avoiding twisting/bending action while lifting is your first line of defense.

What is important for you to achieve is the balancing of both front and back muscles of the trunk. Stretching and strengthening the muscles is important, along with maintaining good posture. Observing the way you sit and stand by keeping the low back and pelvis balanced is another way to prevent the psoas muscles from tightening or weakening.

An easy way to stretch the psoas is to lunge forward with one leg in front and straightening the back leg behind you stretching the front of the back leg. A good way to strengthen the psoas and hip flexors is to do abdominal crunches with your legs off the ground. With proper stretching and strengthening, your back will stay balanced, and you are more likely to keep your psoas silent.

BODY BRIEFS, June, 1994

POWER STANCE

According to Roger Sperry, Ph.D, Nobel Prize recipient, 'better than 90% of the energy output of the brain is used in relating to the physical body in its gravitational field. The more mechanically distorted a person is, the less energy available for thinking, metabolism and healing." In other words, **poor posture** can stress your neck, back, legs, feet and your brain. It can cause constant tiredness, discomfort, headaches, poor breathing, lowcred resistance to disease, and poor blood flow to the *brain*. Eventually you will see a loss in height, a rounding of the shoulders and upper back degeneration of the spinal column, and spinal nerve stress. Doesn't sound too exciting, does it?

Whether you are aware of it or not, your standing, sitting, walking and sleeping postures all have a profound effect on the musculoskeletal function. For healthy human beings, good posture is a relaxed, comfortable, balanced state which provides you with energy, poise and stability. This balanced state helps you deal effectively against the force of gravity.

Your ideal posture consists of three factors: 1) skeletal structure, 2) soft-tissue integrity, and 3) neurological control. These are elements of health which chiropractic care and exercise prescription deal with every day. First, proper alignment of the vertebral bodies in the spine help to prevent joint dysfunction, which leads to reduced mobility and compromised nerve flow. Second, muscles and fascia should be balanced, in order to avoid chronic shortening and weakening of the connective tissues. An imbalance will show up as spasms, cramping, and straining of the muscles. Third, what controls your ability to stand erect against gravity is a complex interaction of several neurological factors. These include inborn postural reflexes, pain avoidance postures, learned behaviors and acquired habits.

The challenge to you is to find ways to improve your posture with a program of stretching, strengthening and spinal alignment. You must also look at common habit patterns and repetitive movements which create stress and tension in your body. This includes sitting at a computer for hours every day with few or no breaks, poor sleeping positions, and slouching while standing or sitting.

The good news is that good, postural habits can be integrated into your lifestyle with a minimal amount of effort. The bad news is, left to your own negligence, you will shrink and degenerate over time until you are too stiff and fragile to move. The choice is yours. Maintaining a **high** quality of life is a **daily** decision. It means stretching daily, exercising regularly, and getting your spine adjusted every 500 miles. So , is it time for a tune-up?

BODY BRIEFS, October, 1994

SLOUCHING TOWARDS RETIREMENT

Before I moved to California in 1976, I read a book about California called Slouching towards Bethlehem by Joan Didion. She wrote about all the different influences, both good and bad, about the way life was in California. While I have forgotten most of what the book was about, I have not forgotten the title, and have taken poetic license to modify it.

Your mother always told you to stand up straight and not slouch when you sat, but alas, you went ahead and did it the way that felt right to you, and look at you now. Your posture is not the man (and woman) you used to be (ah, yesterday). Why? Because your slouching is the tendency towards *progressive deterioration* - forward head, humped back, tilted pelvis. This means that your normal patterns of activity and movement have become less efficient biomechanically, causing you to use more effort and energy just trying to stay upright.

Your posture reflects how well, or poorly, you resist the constant force of gravity, and how you stand, sit, walk and sleep impacts the normal function of your musculoskeletal system. Even the ancient Greeks saw this and realized that those people who had the best posture tended to be the healthiest.

Think of your body as having four main blocks - the head/neck, torso, pelvis and legs, all stacked on top of each other. There should be an evenness and natural alignment to these blocks when you are standing. If these blocks don't stack up evenly, instead of falling down, as would a child's set of blocks, they create a *strained imbalance*, which equates to aches, pains, spasms, tightness and soreness.

There are reflexes and nerve endings in your bodies, plus opposing muscle groups, which are supposed to help hold you together in a balanced manner. However, when there is *chronic, postural overload* and *repetitive movement* the same way day after day, year after year, you override those reflexes and shorten those muscles until you're standing and walking like Groucho Marx.

So, what to do? Be aware of how you move and stop during the day. Are you standing evenly on both legs, knees unlocked, shoulders relaxed? Are you sitting with your pelvis level, back supported by the chair, head balanced over your shoulders? If not, then it's time you did a postural evaluation on yourself and note what changes you can make. Then, as you head toward retirement, your body will be in good enough shape to enjoy it.

BODY BRIEFS, January, 2001

INDEX

A ankles 33, 35
anterior tibialis muscle 9
arms 15-19, 41-43, 46

B back 20-26, 35, 38, 40-45
biceps muscle 9, 15, 16, 46

C calves 32, 33, 35, 44, 45
Carpal Tunnel Syndrome 16-19, 40, 41, 46
chest 14, 41, 43, 46

D deltoid muscle 9, 14, 16, 40, 43, 46

E erector spinae muscles 9, 20-26, 35, 38, 40-45
extension 22, 23, 36-38, 40, 41, 43, 44

F face 12, 39
fascia 8
feet 32, 33
flexion 22, 24, 35-37, 40

G gastrocnemius muscle 9, 32, 33, 44, 45
gluteal muscle 9, 27, 28, 34, 36, 40

H hamstring 9, 32, 44, 45
hands 16-19, 40, 46
hips 27, 28, 35, 37

I iliocostalis muscle 9, 22-27, 36-38, 41
iliotibial band 9, 26

J/K

L legs 29-32, 44, 45
levator scapula muscle 9, 11, 12, 14, 16, 39, 46

M/N neck 10-12, 39, 46

O office stretches 40, 41

P pectoralis 14, 16, 41, 43, 46
pelvis 27, 28, 35-38, 40
piriformis 9, 27, 37, 38, 40
plantar fascia 9, 32, 40
popliteus 9, 31, 32, 44, 45
posterio tibialis 9, 32, 44, 45
Posture (efficient sitting) 47

Q quadratus lumborum 9, 22-28, 35-37, 38, 40-45
quadriceps muscles 9, 30, 41, 43-45

R rhomboid muscles 9, 14, 22, 35, 43
rotation stretches 25, 35-37, 40, 42, 44

S shoulders 14-16, 40, 43, 46
soleus 9, 32, 44, 45
sternocleidomastoid 9, 11, 12, 16, 39
supraspinatus 9, 11, 14, 39, 42, 43, 46

T thighs 30, 31, 41, 43-45
trapezius muscles 9, 11, 12, 14, 16, 39, 42, 43, 46
triceps 9, 15, 46

U/V

W wake-up stretches 34
waves (wrist stretch) 19
wrist 16-19, 40, 41, 46

ABOUT THE AUTHOR

Benjamin Griffes has been in the health care field for the past 20 years. He was trained as a Hellerwork practitioner in 1981, earned a Master's Degree in Physical Education in 1986, and completed his Doctor of Chiropractic degree in 1990. He has written numerous articles, given lectures, and taught classes on health and fitness for the past 18 years. For the past three years he has taught a weekly stretching class near his office in Tarzana, CA. He coaches youth soccer and club track and field, plus runs and mountain bikes for health and pleasure. He lives with his wife and three children in Thousand Oaks, CA.

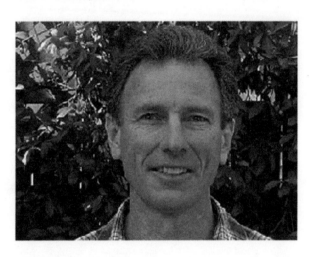

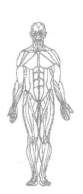